Simplified Solution Approach

To ENDOMETRIOSIS

Unlocking Natural Healing: A Comprehensive Guide to Reclaiming Your Well-being And Strategies for Overcoming Health Challenges

Dr QUENTIN GLYN

Table Of Contents

CHAPTER ONE 6

Endometriosis 6

An Outline Of Endometriosis: 7

Historical Background: 9

CHAPTER TWO 12

Knowing What Endometriosis Is..........12

The Pathogenesis Of Endometriosis:.12

Hazardous Elements: 14

Typical Symptoms:.........................15

CHAPTER THREE 20

Methods Of Diagnosis 20

Clinical Assessment:......................20

Imaging Methodologies: 22

Diagnostic Laparoscopy: 23

CHAPTER FOUR 26

Conventional Therapy Methods 26

Drugs: 26

Hormonal Treatments: 28

Surgical Procedures: 29

Simplified Method Of Solving: 31

CHAPTER FIVE 34

Lifestyle And Holistic Methods For
Treating Endometriosis..........................34

Diet And Nutrition:...............................34

Physical Activity And Exercise: 36

Handling Stress:...................................37

CHAPTER SIX.....................................40

Alternative Medicine 40

Acupuncture..41

Herbal Remedies:................................42

Mind-Body Methodologies:...............44

CHAPTER SEVEN 48

Views From Patients............................48

Patient Perspectives: 48

Personal Narratives: 50

Coping Techniques: 51

Support Systems: 53

CHAPTER EIGHT 56

New Advances In Research And
Innovation 56

Current Study Results: 57

Potential Treatments In The Near
Future: 59

Technological Progress: 61

CHAPTER NINE 64

Education And Advocacy 64

Increasing Conscience: 64

Advocacy For Patients: 67

Initiatives For Education: 68

Conclusion 71

An Overview Of The Main Points 72

Motivation For Individuals Affected: 74

A Request For Further Research And
Assistance: 76

THE END 79

CHAPTER ONE
Endometriosis

Endometriosis is a complicated and often excruciating medical disorder that affects people who are born with a female reproductive system. This condition develops when endometrial tissue, which resembles the lining of the uterus, grows outside the organ.

Although the precise etiology of endometriosis is still unknown, millions of people worldwide are impacted by this serious health issue for women. The definition and fundamentals of endometriosis, its frequency, and the historical background that has influenced our comprehension of this illness will all be covered in this conversation.

An Outline Of Endometriosis:

Definition and Overview: Endometriosis is a gynecological condition marked by tissue outside of the uterus that resembles endometrial tissue. This tissue may grow on the outside of the uterus, the fallopian tubes, and the ovaries, among other pelvic organs. The misplaced tissue in endometriosis cannot leave the body like the normal endometrial tissue, which sheds after menstruation. This may have an effect on fertility as it causes discomfort, inflammation, and the development of adhesions and scar tissue.

While endometriosis symptoms may vary greatly from person to person, they often include pelvic discomfort, infertility, painful menstruation (dysmenorrhea), and pain during sexual activity. Urinary and gastrointestinal problems might sometimes be experienced by endometriosis patients.

Prevalence and Effects on Women's Health: Roughly 10% of people who are of reproductive age have endometriosis, making it a common disorder. It is one of the main causes of infertility and persistent pelvic discomfort. Beyond only its physical manifestations, endometriosis has an influence on relationships, mental health, and quality of life.

Due to the chronic nature of the illness and the difficulties in diagnosing it, diagnosis and treatment are often delayed. The emotional toll of dealing with a painful, long-term illness may exacerbate anxiety and despair, which emphasizes the need for an all-encompassing strategy to manage endometriosis.

Historical Background:

Over time, knowledge and awareness of endometriosis have changed. In the past, the illness's symptoms were often disregarded, and those who suffered from it were not acknowledged. Insufficient knowledge and comprehension resulted in postponed diagnosis and restricted therapeutic alternatives.

The late 19th and early 20th centuries saw the publication of the first thorough accounts of endometriosis. In spite of this, it took many decades for doctors to recognize endometriosis as a real medical issue. The widespread perception that pelvic discomfort was a typical aspect of menstruation impeded efforts to identify and treat the effects of endometriosis.

In recent decades, advances in laparoscopic surgery, medical imaging, and research approaches have led to a better understanding of endometriosis. Better diagnosis methods, earlier therapies, and a more caring approach to treating the condition's psychological and physical symptoms are all results of more knowledge.

To sum up, endometriosis is a complex illness that has a significant effect on women's health. To effectively diagnose, treat, and assist those impacted by this difficult disorder, it is essential to comprehend its definition, prevalence, and historical background. Technological and medical developments are still influencing the treatment of endometriosis, but they also provide hope for better results and a higher standard of living for people who have the disease.

CHAPTER TWO

Knowing What Endometriosis Is

A medical disorder known as endometriosis is defined by the formation of endometrial-like tissue outside of the uterus. The ovaries, fallopian tubes, uterine exteriors, and other pelvic organs all include this misdirected tissue. In extreme situations, it may even spread beyond the pelvic area.

The Pathogenesis Of Endometriosis:

Though its actual etiology is unknown, a number of ideas have been proposed to try to explain the disease's progression. Retrograde menstruation is a well-known notion in which endometrial cells seen in menstrual blood travel backward into the pelvic cavity rather than out of the body. Endometriotic lesions may then develop as a result of these cells adhering to the surfaces and organs of the pelvis.

Immune system dysfunction is thought to be involved as well, as the body may not be able to get rid of endometrial cells that aren't in the right position. Furthermore thought to be possible causes of endometriosis development include hereditary variables, hormone abnormalities, and environmental factors.

Adhesions and scar tissue may develop when endometrial tissue expands outside the uterus. In some situations, this may cause discomfort and infertility as well as cause the pelvic anatomy to become distorted.

Hazardous Elements:

The following variables may make endometriosis more likely to develop:

1. Family History: The risk may be increased if a close relative—such as a mother or sister—has endometriosis.

2. Menstrual History: Prolonged periods, early menstrual onset, and short menstrual cycles may raise the risk.

3. Obstruction of Menstrual Flow: A closed hymen or cervical stenosis are two conditions that might obstruct the regular flow of menstrual blood.

4. Reproductive History: Women who are infertile or have never given birth may be at a greater risk.

5. Autoimmune Disorders: Endometriosis risk may be higher in conditions when the immune system is weakened or malfunctioning.

6. Ethnicity: Although the exact causes of this are unknown, studies indicate that endometriosis may be more prevalent in women from certain ethnic backgrounds.

Typical Symptoms:

Endometriosis symptoms may vary greatly from person to person, and some people may not have any symptoms at all. Typical indications and manifestations include:

1. Pelvic Pain: The most common symptom, pelvic pain may be minor or quite severe. Often, the discomfort becomes worse throughout the menstrual cycle.

2. Dysmenorrhea, or painful menstruation: Women who have endometriosis often have excruciating cramps throughout their periods.

3. Intense Feeling: Suffering during or after a sexual encounter is a typical sign.

4. urine or Bowel Movement discomfort: Endometriosis, particularly during menstruation, may result in discomfort during urine or bowel movements.

5. Prolonged Menstrual Bleeding: Women who have endometriosis may have prolonged menstrual bleeding.

6. Infertility: One major factor contributing to infertility in women is endometriosis. The reproductive organs' ability to function normally may be impacted by adhesions and scar tissue.

7. Fatigue: A general sense of being poorly and weariness may be caused by several symptoms, including chronic pain.

In conclusion, early identification and successful treatment of endometriosis depend on an awareness of the pathophysiology, risk factors, and typical symptoms of the condition. Prompt action may reduce symptoms, enhance quality of life, and help those who are trying to conceive by addressing reproductive issues.

It is recommended that you speak with a healthcare provider if you have any of these symptoms in order to get an accurate diagnosis and customized treatment recommendations.

CHAPTER THREE
Methods Of Diagnosis

A medical disorder known as endometriosis occurs when endometrial tissue, which resembles the lining of the uterus, develops outside of it. This illness may result in infertility problems and severe discomfort. Making an accurate diagnosis of endometriosis is essential for prompt symptom alleviation and therapy. In most cases, laparoscopic diagnosis is combined with imaging methods and clinical assessment in the diagnostic procedure.

Clinical Assessment:

1. Health Background:

- Symptom Assessment: Detailed conversation on the patient's complaints, including infertility, pelvic discomfort, dysmenorrhea (painful menstruation), and dyspareunia (pain during sexual activity).

• Menstrual History: Comprehensive details on the length, flow, and abnormalities of a woman's menstrual cycle.

2. Physical Assessment:

• Pelvic Exam: Palpation of the pelvic area to look for lumps, sore spots, or irregularities.

• Bimanual Exam: A two-handed pelvic examination used to evaluate the pelvic organs' size, form, and motion.

Imaging Methodologies:

1. Ultrasonography:

• Transvaginal Ultrasound (TVUS): Deep infiltrating endometriosis (DIE) and ovarian endometriomas may be detected using this method, which entails inserting an ultrasound probe into the vagina to provide a more comprehensive view of pelvic tissues.

• Abdominal Ultrasound: This non-invasive method may evaluate pelvic tissues and identify bigger endometriotic cysts on the ovaries.

2. MRIs, or magnetic resonance imaging:

• Pelvic MRI: Offers finely detailed pictures of pelvic tissues, assisting in the detection of adhesions, deep infiltrating endometriosis, and involvement of adjacent structures such as the bladder or intestine.

3. CT (Computerized Tomography) Scan:

• Pelvic CT Scan: Although less frequent than MRI, CT scans may be used to assess the degree of illness and find endometriotic cysts.

Diagnostic Laparoscopy:

1. Reasons to consider a laparoscopy:

• Gold Standard: Because of its accuracy, laparoscopy is regarded as the gold standard for endometriosis diagnosis.

• Unexplained Pelvic discomfort: When other diagnostic techniques fail to explain pelvic discomfort, laparoscopy is often advised.

• Infertility: Laparoscopy may detect and cure endometriosis in situations of infertility that cannot be explained.

2. Method:

• Minimally Invasive: Laparoscopy requires a few tiny incisions through which a thin, illuminated tube (laparoscope) is placed. This allows the surgeon to see the organs located in the pelvis.

• Tissue Biopsy: To confirm the existence of endometriotic lesions, tissue samples may be taken for a biopsy during a laparoscopy.

3. Setting:

- Revised American Society for Reproductive Medicine (rASRM) Staging: Depending on the size, location, and severity of lesions, endometriosis is often staged during a laparoscopy. Treatment choices are guided in part by staging.

In summary:

A thorough diagnostic process for endometriosis combines imaging methods, clinical assessment, and, if required, surgical diagnosis. Although non-invasive imaging techniques and clinical assessment provide useful data, laparoscopy is still required for precise diagnosis and staging. For those with endometriosis, an early and precise diagnosis allows for prompt intervention, symptom management, and better results.

CHAPTER FOUR
Conventional Therapy Methods

A medical disorder known as endometriosis occurs when endometrial, or uterine, tissue begins to proliferate outside of the uterus. This illness may cause discomfort and result in a number of problems. Medications, hormonal therapy, and surgical procedures are often used in conjunction with traditional treatment methods for endometriosis. Let's examine each of these strategies in further detail:

Drugs:

1. Pain Management:

• Nonsteroidal Anti-Inflammatory Drugs (NSAIDs): Ibuprofen and other similar medications can lessen endometriosis-related pain and inflammation.

• Acetaminophen: For pain relief, it could be advised.

2. Hormonal Supplements:

• Birth Control Pills: Oral contraceptives help lessen endometriosis discomfort and control menstrual periods.

• Gonadotropin-releasing hormone (GnRH) Antagonists and Agonists: These medications cause a transient menopausal state by inhibiting the release of estrogen. They may lessen the symptoms brought on by the expansion of endometrial tissue.

• Progestin Therapy: Progestin, a synthetic version of progesterone, may lessen symptoms and assist in regulating the development of endometrial tissue.

3. Danazol:

• This synthetic medication reduces endometriosis symptoms by suppressing ovulation and inducing a pseudo-menopausal state.

Hormonal Treatments:

1. Hormonal contraceptives combined:

• Estrogen and progestin-containing birth control tablets, patches, or vaginal rings help balance menstrual cycles and reduce symptoms.

2. Progestin Treatment:

• Endometriosis symptoms may be managed with progestin-only contraceptives, including injections, implants, or intrauterine devices.

3. Antagonists and Agonists of GnRH:

• These medications cause a menopausal-like condition by suppressing the synthesis of estrogen. Because of the possible adverse effects, they are often taken for a brief time only.

Surgical Procedures:

1. Laparoscopy:

• To see and perhaps remove endometrial tissue growths, a tiny incision is used to introduce a thin, illuminated tube during this minimally invasive surgical technique.

2. Laparoscopy:

• To remove bigger endometrial growths or cysts, conventional open surgery may be required in more severe situations.

3. Hysterectomy:

• Removing the uterus (and maybe the ovaries) may be an option if all other therapies have failed and the patient does not want to maintain fertility.

4. Surgery via Excision:

• This entails excising or eliminating endometrial tissue while leaving the surrounding, healthy tissue intact. It is regarded as a more sophisticated and successful surgical technique.

Simplified Method Of Solving:

1. Early Diagnosis:

• Prompt diagnosis is essential to efficient treatment. Women who have symptoms such as infertility, unpleasant periods, or pelvic discomfort should contact a doctor.

2. Tailored Care Programs:

• It is crucial to customize therapy regimens based on the unique symptoms, age, and goal for fertility preservation of each patient.

3. Combination Counseling:

• Using both hormonal therapy and prescription drugs together may often result in greater symptom management than either strategy alone.

4. Patient Instruction:

In order to make an educated choice, people must be informed about the nature of endometriosis, available treatments, and any adverse effects.

5. Multidisciplinary Method:

• In complicated circumstances, gynecologists, pain management specialists, and fertility specialists working together may provide a holistic treatment plan.

In conclusion, treating endometriosis holistically and individually, with the use of hormone therapy, pharmaceuticals, and surgery where necessary, may help patients control their symptoms and enhance their quality of life. An effective treatment approach requires frequent follow-ups and open communication between patients and healthcare professionals.

CHAPTER FIVE

Lifestyle And Holistic Methods For Treating Endometriosis

Diet And Nutrition:

Anti-inflammatory Diet: Managing the inflammation brought on by endometriosis may be facilitated by using an anti-inflammatory diet. This entails eating less pro-inflammatory foods like processed carbohydrates and saturated fats and increasing consumption of foods high in omega-3 fatty acids, which are present in walnuts, flaxseeds, and fatty fish.

Foods High in Fiber: Consuming a diet rich in fiber, which comes from fruits, vegetables, and whole grains, might help maintain hormonal balance, improve digestive health, and perhaps lessen the symptoms of endometriosis.

Plant-Based Diet: A plant-based diet has been associated with symptom improvements for some people. Antioxidants and phytochemicals included in plant-based diets are often abundant and may promote general health.

Limiting Alcohol and Caffeine: As these drugs may worsen inflammation and upset hormonal balance, reducing alcohol and caffeine intake may be beneficial for those with endometriosis.

Physical Activity And Exercise:

Low-Impact Exercise: Without placing too much effort on the body, low-impact workouts like cycling, swimming, or strolling may assist in improving cardiovascular health and decrease stress.

Pilates and yoga are three types of exercise that emphasize strength, flexibility, and relaxation. Certain postures and exercises may alleviate pelvic discomfort and enhance general health.

Aerobic Exercise: Consistent aerobic exercise has been linked to a decrease in inflammation and may help with pain relief. To ascertain the proper amount of exercise for a given situation, speaking with a healthcare provider is essential.

Handling Stress:

Exercises that encourage mindfulness and meditation are beneficial for reducing stress, which is known to aggravate endometriosis symptoms. People who practice mindfulness may manage their discomfort and feel less anxious.

Breathing Techniques: By inducing a relaxation response, deep breathing techniques may help reduce stress and tension in the muscles. There may be advantages to learning and using deep breathing exercises in everyday life.

Good Sleep: Getting enough sleep is essential for maintaining good health. A regular sleep schedule and a calming setting before bed may help improve the quality of sleep, which may have a beneficial effect on endometriosis symptoms.

Although lifestyle changes and holistic treatments cannot treat endometriosis, they may improve general health and perhaps lessen certain symptoms. Endometriosis patients must collaborate closely with medical specialists to create a customized, all-encompassing treatment plan that may include a mix of pharmaceutical treatments, complementary therapies, and lifestyle changes.

By combining these strategies, endometriosis patients may benefit from a more comprehensive and well-rounded approach to controlling their disease and leading better lives.

CHAPTER SIX
Alternative Medicine

Enhancing general health and controlling endometriosis symptoms are important roles that complementary treatments may play.

It is important to acknowledge that while these methods may provide alleviation for some people, they must be used in conjunction with a thorough treatment regimen and not as an alternative to traditional medical measures.

Before adding complementary treatments to your regimen, always get advice from your doctor.

Acupuncture

Definition: Acupuncture is a traditional Chinese medicine that stimulates the flow of Qi, or energy, by inserting tiny needles into certain body sites. Acupuncture is thought to help balance the body's energy and lessen discomfort in the setting of endometriosis.

Mechanism of Action: Acupuncture may improve blood circulation and trigger the body's natural analgesics, endorphins, to be released. It is also believed to have an impact on the neurological system, lowering inflammation and modifying pain signals.

Evidence: Acupuncture may help reduce discomfort associated with endometriosis and enhance the quality of life, according to some research. To definitively confirm its effectiveness, additional study is necessary.

Acupuncture is usually regarded as safe when administered by a qualified and certified professional. To make sure acupuncture fits into your entire treatment plan, it's important to let your healthcare practitioner know about your desire to investigate it.

Herbal Remedies:

Definition: Using plant-based materials to treat certain health issues and enhance health is known as herbal medicine. Certain herbs are thought to have anti-inflammatory and hormone-balancing effects in relation to endometriosis.

Common medicines: Turmeric (curcumin), ginger, chamomile, and Chinese medicines like danshen and licorice root are a few examples of herbs that are used to control endometriosis.

Mechanism of Action: In addition to possibly influencing hormonal balance, herbs have the ability to affect the immune system and reduce inflammation. It's crucial to remember that there is little scientific proof of herbal medicine's effectiveness in treating endometriosis and that each person will react differently.

Considerations: Before using herbal medicines, speak with a licensed herbalist or healthcare professional. Certain herbs may interact with pharmaceuticals or be contraindicated. It is important to take herbal medication carefully and under supervision.

Mind-Body Methodologies:

Definition: Mind-body approaches are methods that emphasize how the mind and body work together to support general health. Techniques for relaxation and stress management are often highlighted in relation to endometriosis.

Examples of mind-body practices that may be helpful include mindfulness meditation, yoga, deep breathing exercises, and progressive muscle relaxation.

Mechanism of Action: Mind-body therapies try to lower stress levels, which may worsen endometriosis symptoms. These techniques may also aid in controlling pain perception and enhancing mental health in general.

Evidence: Although studies on mind-body therapies for endometriosis are still in progress, they seem to have the potential to enhance pain relief and overall quality of life.

It should be noted that mind-body methods are usually safe and well-tolerated. It is vital to choose practices that align with your own inclinations and comfort zone. Over time, implementing these methods into a regular practice can have cumulative advantages.

To sum up, complementary treatments like herbal medicine, acupuncture, and mind-body methods may be important parts of an all-encompassing strategy for controlling endometriosis. Individual reactions can differ, however, so these strategies should be included in a thorough treatment plan along with traditional medical measures and continued contact with healthcare professionals. When thinking about complementary treatments, always get expert advice to make sure they meet your unique requirements and objectives for health.

CHAPTER SEVEN
Views From Patients

Millions of women worldwide suffer from endometriosis, a complicated and sometimes incapacitating medical illness. For a holistic approach to treating endometriosis, it is as important to understand patient views, personal experiences, coping mechanisms, and support networks as it is to implement medical therapies.

Patient Perspectives: Developing practical remedies requires an understanding of endometriosis from the patient's point of view. Patients often deal with mental discomfort, exhaustion, and chronic pain.

It is essential to understand how it affects their relationships, everyday life, and mental health in order to create comprehensive treatment strategies.

• Obstacles Patients Face:

• Chronic discomfort: A lot of people with endometriosis have pelvic discomfort that doesn't go away, making it difficult for them to work, socialize, and go about their everyday lives.

• Diagnostic Delays: Patients' emotional distress is exacerbated and frustration is increased when the diagnostic process takes longer than expected.

• Mental Health Issues: Anxiety, despair, and feelings of loneliness may result from the emotional strain and the unpredictability of the disease.

Personal Narratives: Telling one's own tales strengthens bonds with others and encourages empathy. Real-life stories encourage patients to be resilient and hopeful in addition to increasing awareness.

• Powerful Storytelling:

• Diagnosis Journeys: Telling others about the difficulties encountered during diagnosis enables them to better navigate the healthcare system.

• Treatment Experiences: Individualized narratives of diverse treatment modalities provide insightful information to individuals weighing their alternatives.

• Life Beyond Endometriosis: Success stories of people who successfully manage their illness give others hope and motivation.

Coping Techniques: Giving patients coping techniques improves their capacity to handle the psychological and physical effects of endometriosis.

• Pain Reduction Strategies:

• Practicing mindfulness, yoga, and meditation may help manage chronic pain and enhance general well-being.

• Acupuncture and heat treatment are complementary therapies that some patients find helpful.

• Assisting Emotionally:

• Online forums and support groups provide a forum for exchanging insights and counsel.

Patients who are dealing with the emotional difficulties brought on by a chronic disease might benefit from therapy and counseling.

• Alterations to Lifestyle:

• For some people, dietary modifications, such as anti-inflammatory diets, may reduce symptoms.

• Maintaining general health requires striking a balance between exercise and relaxation.

Support Systems: Creating strong support networks is essential to endometriosis patients' overall health.

• Medical Practitioners:

A comprehensive therapeutic method necessitates collaboration between gynecologists, pain experts, and mental health doctors.

• Treatment programs that are tailored to each patient's requirements and preferences are guaranteed by patient-centered care.

• Friends and Family:

• Educating loved ones about endometriosis promotes empathy and support by helping them understand the difficulties sufferers encounter.

• Providing patients with practical help with everyday duties during flare-ups may greatly enhance their quality of life.

• Awareness and Advocacy:

• In order to better the lives of persons who have endometriosis, advocacy organizations are essential in spreading knowledge, pushing for research, and encouraging legislative reforms.

• Raising public knowledge lessens stigma and promotes a culture that is more understanding and kind.

In summary, a method that simplifies solutions for endometriosis has to take into account the viewpoints of patients by using support networks, coping mechanisms, and personal narratives. We may strive toward a more inclusive and functional framework that enables people to live better, healthier lives despite the difficulties presented by endometriosis by accepting the complex character of this illness.

CHAPTER EIGHT

New Advances In Research And Innovation

The development of endometrial-like tissue outside the uterus is a complicated and often debilitating disorder known as endometriosis. Affected persons experience discomfort, inflammation, and problems with fertility.

As the field's research continues, there have been significant advancements in our knowledge of the underlying causes of endometriosis, along with novel techniques for diagnosis and therapy. With an emphasis on recent study results, potential future treatments, and technology breakthroughs, let's examine the field's newest discoveries and research from this perspective.

Current Study Results:

Genetic and Molecular Understanding: Lately, research has focused on the genetic and molecular aspects of endometriosis. In order to shed light on possible susceptibility factors, researchers have discovered certain genetic markers linked to an increased chance of acquiring the illness.

Immune System Involvement: A great deal of research has been done on how the immune system is involved in endometriosis. In order to create targeted therapeutics, it is essential to comprehend the interaction between endometriotic lesions and the immune system. Immune dysregulation may have a role in the development and survival of endometriotic tissue, according to research.

Biomarkers for Early Detection: Research is being done to find trustworthy biomarkers for endometriosis early diagnosis and detection. The speed and precision of diagnosis might be greatly increased by the introduction of non-invasive diagnostic instruments like blood testing and imaging methods.

Microbiome and Endometriosis: Research on the connection between the microbiome and endometriosis is only being started.

Gaining insight into how the microbiome affects the onset and course of the illness might lead to the development of novel treatment approaches.

Potential Treatments In The Near Future:

Immunomodulatory treatments: Research is being done on immunomodulatory treatments in light of the expanding knowledge about the role of the immune system. The goal of these therapies is to control immunological reactions and maybe stop endometriosis from progressing further.

Targeted Therapies: Specific molecular targets linked to endometriosis have been identified thanks to developments in precision medicine. More precise targeted medicines that address the underlying processes are being researched, including hormonal and non-hormonal alternatives.

Stem Cell Treatment: Endometriosis stem cell treatment is becoming more and more popular. Regenerative therapy techniques have promise due to the capacity of stem cells to heal damaged tissue and regulate the inflammatory environment.

Personalized medicine: Current research aims to customize treatment plans according to a patient's genetic composition and unique illness features. Personalized medicine may reduce adverse effects and increase the effectiveness of therapy.

Technological Progress:

Artificial Intelligence in Diagnosis: To diagnose endometriosis more precisely and effectively, AI is being used to evaluate medical imaging, such as MRI and ultrasound scans. Algorithms that use machine learning may help detect minute symptoms of the illness that conventional analysis would miss.

Telemedicine and Remote Monitoring: By integrating telemedicine, patients may get specialist treatment more easily by having remote consultations and patient monitoring. For those with endometriosis, who may have trouble getting healthcare services, this is very helpful.

Surgical Innovations: To improve the accuracy and effectiveness of endometriosis operations, less invasive surgical methods, such as robotic-assisted treatments, are being developed. The goal of these developments is to shorten healing periods and enhance patient outcomes.

Drug Delivery Systems: To increase medicine efficacy while reducing adverse effects, innovations in drug delivery systems, such as targeted drug delivery or sustained-release implants, are being investigated.

In summary, there has been steady progress in our knowledge of endometriosis at the genetic, molecular, and immune levels, making the field's landscape dynamic.

Technological advancements and promising therapeutics have the potential to completely change how endometriosis is diagnosed and treated, giving those living with this difficult ailment hope for better results and a higher quality of life.

CHAPTER NINE

Education And Advocacy

Endometriosis is a multifaceted and often disabling illness affecting the endometrium, the tissue lining the uterus. It may affect millions of people globally and result in discomfort, infertility, and a host of other symptoms. In order to combat endometriosis, help people who are impacted, and foster a greater knowledge of the illness among the general public, advocacy, and education are essential.

Increasing Conscience:

1. Public Ads:

• Public awareness efforts must be launched in order to educate the general public about endometriosis. This may happen via a variety of media, including print materials, radio, television, and social media.

• Using well-known people, celebrities, and influencers to expand the audience for awareness campaigns may aid in drawing in public interest.

2. Local Occasions:

• Putting up community gatherings, lectures, and workshops to provide people a forum to discuss their endometriosis experiences promotes a feeling of belonging and solidarity.

Encouraging people to seek assistance may be achieved by working with medical experts to organize information sessions on symptoms, diagnosis, and available treatments.

3. The month of endometriosis awareness worldwide:

• Setting aside certain months for concentrated awareness campaigns, like March (Endometriosis Awareness Month), might have a significant worldwide influence.

• During this month, endometriosis is made more visible by encouraging local communities, organizations, and people to take part in events like walks, fundraising drives, and educational seminars.

Advocacy For Patients:

1. Support Teams:

• Creating and promoting endometriosis support groups gives people a forum for exchanging stories, coping mechanisms, and emotional support.

• These organizations are accessible to everyone, no matter where they live, since they can be found both online and offline.

2. Advocate for Laws:

• Promoting laws that address the particular difficulties experienced by those who have endometriosis, such as easier access to healthcare, insurance for required treatments, and accommodations at work.

• Working with legislators to increase public knowledge of endometriosis's effects on both people and society as a whole.

3. Advocating for medical care:

• Working together with medical specialists to make sure that procedures are in line with the most recent findings and guidelines for the diagnosis and management of endometriosis.

• Fighting for additional funding for research to learn more about the causes of endometriosis, provide better treatments, and find a cure.

Initiatives For Education:

1. Curriculum in Schools:

• Including instructional modules in the school curriculum about reproductive health and illnesses, such as endometriosis, may assist in increasing youth awareness.

• Offering educational resources to parents, educators, and students guarantees a thorough knowledge and management of endometriosis.

2. Training for Healthcare Providers:

• Providing healthcare workers with specific training to improve their understanding of endometriosis symptoms, diagnosis, and available treatments.

• Promoting the use of a multidisciplinary team to treat endometriosis, including gynecologists, pain management experts, mental health specialists, and other pertinent specialists.

3. Web-Based Resources:

• Creating and maintaining current and accurate online materials regarding endometriosis that are readily accessible, such as webpages, webinars, and videos.

• Working together with respectable medical organizations and institutes to guarantee the veracity and correctness of the data provided.

In conclusion, a thorough approach to endometriosis includes advocating for change and educating the public in addition to expanding medical research and treatment alternatives. Individuals with endometriosis may obtain better treatment by increasing knowledge, offering support, and fostering understanding. Additionally, society at large should endeavor to remove the stigma associated with this often misdiagnosed ailment.

Conclusion

Millions of people worldwide are impacted by the complicated and difficult ailment known as endometriosis, which calls for a comprehensive but straightforward approach to treatment. Let's review the main ideas that have been covered in this method, provide some consolation to those impacted, and make a request for further study and assistance.

An Overview Of The Main Points

1. Early Diagnosis and Detection: Early diagnosis of endometriosis depends on the ability to identify its telltale signs and symptoms. Faster diagnosis and intervention may result from increased knowledge among the general population and healthcare professionals.

2. Multidisciplinary Approach: Gynecologists, pain experts, surgeons, and mental health specialists must work together to manage endometriosis. Working together may improve the overall health and treatment that people with endometriosis get.

3. Patient Education: It's critical to provide endometriosis patients with knowledge and empowerment. Patients may actively engage in their care and make educated choices if they are informed about the ailment, available treatments, and lifestyle modifications.

4. Holistic Treatment Modalities: Traditional medical treatments may be enhanced by using holistic methods such as exercise, diet modifications, and alternative therapies. A holistic approach promotes complete well-being by taking into account the mental, emotional, and physical elements of the person.

5. Developments in Medical Research: Finding a cure for endometriosis and

creating more effective treatments will need sustained investment in medical research. Research projects that get funding and support may lead to discoveries into the underlying causes and workings of the ailment.

6. Advocacy for Policy Changes: Attempts to change healthcare policy via advocacy may result in better insurance coverage, research funding, and care accessibility. The endometriosis community as a whole may influence improvements in healthcare systems across the world.

Motivation For Individuals Affected:

It is important for those dealing with endometriosis to keep in mind that they are not alone in their struggles. Though the path may be challenging, there is hope and assistance accessible. Look for groups where people discuss their experiences, provide guidance, and offer emotional support—both online and off. Recall that self-care is essential, and that consulting with medical specialists who specialize in endometriosis may have a substantial impact.

It's important to recognize the fortitude and tenacity shown by endometriosis patients. Your stories inspire constructive change and help raise awareness of the illness. In the quest for improved care and understanding, remember to appreciate tiny accomplishments, have patience with yourself, and realize that your voice counts.

A Request For Further Research And Assistance:

There is still more work to be done, even though endometriosis is now better understood and treated. The following activities may support current initiatives:

1. Encourage Research Initiatives: Push for more public and private financing for endometriosis research. To speed up the creation of novel therapies, promote cooperation between academic institutions, pharmaceutical corporations, and researchers.

2. Raise Awareness: Keep spreading the word about endometriosis online, at your workplace, and in your community.

Education may help break down stereotypes, lessen stigma, and promote understanding.

3. Participate in Advocacy: Become a member of or provide assistance to endometriosis advocacy organizations. These organizations often have a significant impact in lobbying for enhanced funding for research, better healthcare practices, and regulatory reforms.

4. Promote Honest and Open Discussions: Encourage candid and open discussions around endometriosis. Tear down the walls of silence and invite people to talk about their experiences. This may lessen the isolation that is often linked to the illness and help create a community that is supportive.

In summary, we may strive toward a simpler solution approach to endometriosis by combining early identification, a multidisciplinary approach, patient education, holistic treatment modalities, improvements in medical research, campaigning for governmental reforms, and continued support for individuals afflicted. By working together, we can significantly enhance the lives of those who suffer from endometriosis and forward the larger objective of discovering a treatment.

THE END